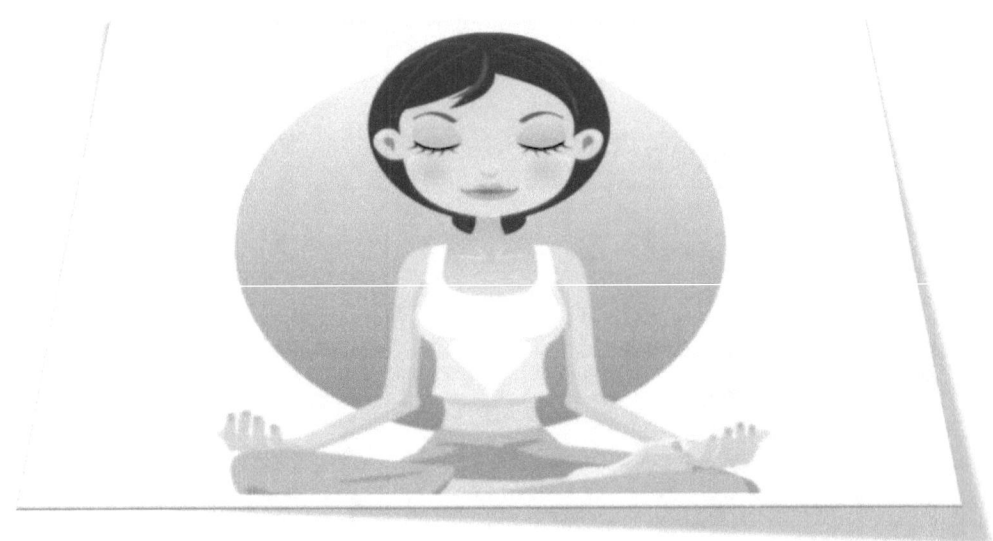

Yoga: Linking the Mind, Body, and Soul.

Do you want to know the benefits of yoga? Then you have purchased the right book. I want to thank you and congratulate you for downloading the book, *"The Beginner's Guide to Yoga"*.

Most beginners view Yoga as a fast and easy way to achieve their goal of losing weight. Others see it as a simple recreational activity that would make them relax and forget all the stress of day-to-day life. But what most people do not realize is the fact that Yoga is more than what was mentioned. And for a beginner to fully utilize the benefits of Yoga, it is necessary to know what it really is and determine if it can give you what you need for a balance life. When you truly practice yoga, you will learn to link your mind, body and soul in harmony.

Given the fact stated, it is then the responsibility of a Yoga Practitioner to understand the roots of Yoga. This book will first and foremost inform you about its history. You will then be able to see what is the main purpose of the existence of Yoga and where it acquired all the knowledge it uses to channel positive energy to a person's life.

It is also necessary to know that Yoga is influenced by eastern religious practices. But it does not mean you will be converting into their faith by practicing Yoga. Still, it is best to understand these religions in order to advance your understanding what really is the goal of Yoga itself.

Once knowing the basics information of what Yoga is, then you will be ready to prepare yourself on what you need for each Yoga session. You will be informed about the necessities and what you do not really need every time you hit the mat.

Finally, this will not become a beginner's guide if you will not learn about a few basic Yoga poses. The poses chosen are suitable for a beginner especially for those people starting out with lesser body flexibility. But all these poses will guarantee that once you practice and master them, you will be on your way to become an expert Yoga practitioner.

You need to remember though that this is just a guide. It will not be able to help you out if you are not determined yourself. But once you learn the purpose of Yoga itself, determination will become second nature to you along with other benefits that Yoga will bring into your life.

Thanks again for downloading this book, I hope you enjoy it!

-MARY PETERS

Table of Contents

What is Yoga?

It would be hard to pinpoint one exact definition for the term "Yoga" since it varies greatly from culture to culture. But the idea that unites all the variations of Yoga is the belief that anyone who is able to practice it properly and consistently will achieve a desired transformation of the mind and body.

Yoga is reinvigoration for the body, mind and soul. Its official meaning is 'union' and the art form certainly takes on great obstacles to unite the three parts of our body. When this union occurs, however, it is very magical and inspiring to say the least. It takes a great power of the mind to conquer some of the moves of yoga, but with a focus on the mind rather than the matter at hand, the mazing moves can be performed and an individual can find an inner peace and calmness they never before knew existed.

The cultures that use Yoga as a way for this transformation were able to develop their own schools that teach their own ways of Yoga. Each has unique approach that is base on their religious belief. They also have their own ways and goals in practicing Yoga but all simply leads to the desire of achieving enlightenment of the mind and the purification of the body.

This belief unfortunately have been gift wrapped into a desirable package and is then presented to the western culture mostly as a way of weight control. In a sense this could be one of the goals of Yoga but practicing for this purpose alone is not enough as motivation to practice its real essence. A beginning Yoga practitioner such as you then must understand this essence first before trying to see what Yoga school fits your personality best or if Yoga fits you at all.

A. Brief History

Yoga is said to have originated in India even before its Vedic tradition started. But its full development only began around the 6th century BCE. From there the various traditional schools developed in parallel with each other started developing to what they are today.

Yoga was then introduced to the west following the same traditions the gurus used in the Yoga's place of origin. It was only until the 1980s that Yoga was transformed by popular culture to the popular system of physical exercise.

The term "Yoga" itself has multiple meanings and origin. It is said that it was first meant to denote the "yoking" of the horse and its rider. Meaning the rider must be able to be one with the horse to be able to control it freely as if part of the rider's body. It was also said that "yoga" relates to the control of the chariot that depicts the similar concept.

Later, the "yoking" term of Yoga was developed to being one with your own physically, mentally and spiritually. In a sense it has a similar concept to the control of the horse and the chariot and most likely would require the same amount of discipline.

B. The Goal

The word "liberation" is often associated as the main goal of Yoga. But again, the exact meaning of this term differs from what school you are following as a Yoga practitioner. Sometimes it means the liberation of the self from any worldly desires and thus achieving enlightenment. Or it may sometimes mean the liberation of the self from the bondage of the past that burdens a person to move on.

It can be argued though that Yoga technically has five principal purposes. The first one is utilizing Yoga as a disciplined method of achieving a goal. This means that a practitioner must have a specific goal in mind and thus use the teachings of the Yoga school to achieve this goal. This usually involves not only physical workouts but also mental and spiritual exercises.

The second purpose of Yoga is its use as a control for both body and the mind. Control over this two aspects aims to achieve balance and maintain it. Which many believes that it is a good way to achieve satisfaction in life.

Yoga also has the third purpose of being a journey of self-realization. It can become a way to analyze yourself in terms of your perception of the world. Technically, this can become the first goal of the beginning Yoga practitioner such as you before embarking on the other purposes. Knowing your true self first will eventually lead to the utilization of the other purposes of Yoga in your life.

Fourth, you may use Yoga as a way to expand your consciousness and views of the world. It can be a way for an open mind. It will then lead to becoming more optimistic and perceptive in dealing with various scenarios you may encounter in life.

The fifth and can be said as the ultimate purpose that could unite all schools of Yoga is to achieve omniscience. This is enlightenment or nirvana itself. But it does not mean being able to become a deity. Omniscience here pertains to your complete understanding of the world around you and could be said to be the direct result of the previous purposes mentioned above.

C. Physiology

Now it is necessary for you to understand as well that Yoga revolves around in the belief that a person has three bodies or "sheets". Each part contributes to the overall existence of the person and thus channeling energy properly into these "sheets" must be done in order to achieve the purpose of Yoga practice.

The first sheet is called the "Sthula Sarira" or the physical form of the body that needs to be nurtured physically. This is the body that demands the basic needs of food, clothing and shelter. Technically, this is the part that comes into full contact of the external world around a person.

"Suksma Sarira" is the second body, which is mainly composed of the intellect and other vital energies, which in turn keep the "Sthula Sarira" alive. Alive here means the person is able to function properly in world in terms of proper interaction and communication. "Suksma Sarira" then can be said as the way the person can perceive the world and create a series of decisions that prompts the "Sthula Sarira" to act.

The third body is the "Karana Sarira". It is said to be the cause of how the "Suksma Sarira" perceives the world. It technically creates the reason behind all the actions the previous two bodies will do. It can be directly related to the spirit of the person that can dictate what the mind and the body will do.

Knowing these information should give you now the basic idea what will be your main goal for practicing Yoga. Once you have a clear and unmoving decision what this goal will be, you can then choose what the best Yoga School is for you.

Schools of Yoga (What Fits You Best)

It was already tackled that Yoga technically differs depending on the culture that implements its practice. Although most of the schools you will be reading about can be directly link to religious practices, it must be emphasized once again that following their traditions does not necessarily mean you are converting your belief and religion.

In this sense you must remember the five main purposes of Yoga that was mentioned in the previous chapter. And if you noticed, none of those stated that you would be changing your belief. What true Yoga does for you is to guide you to achieve your goal in life by implementing discipline in your body, mind and spirit.

A. Buddhism

Yoga in Buddhism revolves mostly in meditation practices that aim to the development of the mind. In order to achieve this development, each meditation must session must have a goal to achieve tranquility, concentration, insight and mindfulness. It is believe to be the way to enlightenment or nirvana.

It is correct for you then to assume that most of the techniques implemented in Buddhism involved sitting and staying still. Though there are some other forms that may also be utilized to increase the overall concentration of the practitioner.

If your goal then is a peace of mind then this is the best school for you. You need to understand though that there are some mediation techniques, which involve chanting prayers to allow the practitioner to be more focus on the process.

B. Hinduism

Yoga in Hinduism is divided into four schools and thus four different practices. These are Hatha Yoga, Raja Yoga, Shaivism Yoga, and Tantra Yoga.

Hatha Yoga focuses in the combination of physical and mental strengthening. Each post and technique implemented requires the practitioner to unite the control of the mind with the movement of the body. The sessions will then build both aspects parallel to each other. This means one aspect must wait if the other is not able to cope. This in turn creates harmony in both body and mind if done properly.

Raja Yoga is somewhat similar to its Buddhist counterpart. The main purpose of this school is making the mind still. Its practices then revolve in stopping any perturbation the mind may encounter.

This results to the total isolation of the self and motionless essence during the session. Each technique if done properly can then allow the mind to be empty of any worries and stress and thus promote relaxation.

Shaivism Yoga on the other hand uses techniques to ultimately unite the practitioner with the presence of a deity. It can be related to achieving nirvana in Buddhism and Raja Yoga but the difference is the reason for reaching the state. Shaivism Yoga teaches that to achieve enlightenment a person must be able to become one with the divine existence in contrast with the other schools which technically focuses on self-enlightenment.

Tantra Yoga is technically the combination of the practices of the previous schools mentioned, starting from Buddhism to Shaivism Yoga. It is a combination of meditative practices that and physical exercises that follows the teachings of the previous schools. It can be said to be the school that tries to combine the best practices to achieve similar results.

C. Jainism

Jainism Yoga techniques are similar to the Saivism Yoga since it also aims for the ultimate freedom and salvation of the soul. It also emphasizes the goal of achieving and staying in the state of true freedom, which is purely conscious and free from any form of attachments. A practitioner must then become someone who sees and someone who knows. This means being aware of everything surrounding himself and thus has the ability to accept each situation as it comes.

D. Modern Schools of Wellness

This is most probably the most popular type of Yoga school today. The main goal is to improve the physical condition of the practitioner in terms of trying to remove any health problems and causes of stress. Modern yoga schools are growing like mushrooms almost everywhere.

In a sense it is actually ok to have many modern Yoga schools since you can practically choose any of them to follow. Each of them claims of course that they follow a specific traditional school but usually they package their techniques as a great way to quickly lose weight. This is where the problem occurs.

Technically it is quite fine if your purpose for practicing Yoga is to lose weight since as the first purpose states you must have a goal you want to achieve. But if you believe that doing the postures and exercises alone will help you out to lose weight as most of the modern schools claim, then you are being misled. To understand this we need to circle back to the five purposes of Yoga and the goals of the traditional Yoga schools. It can be concluded then that the physical exercises must be coupled with the mental and spiritual exercise to implement the discipline that Yoga preaches.

If you wish to enroll in modern Yoga schools then be sure to check their methods and their practices first to ensure that you will not be disappointed in the results you expect. You must understand as well that a good modern school will be giving strict guidance not only in physical exercises but also in mental and spiritual conditioning.

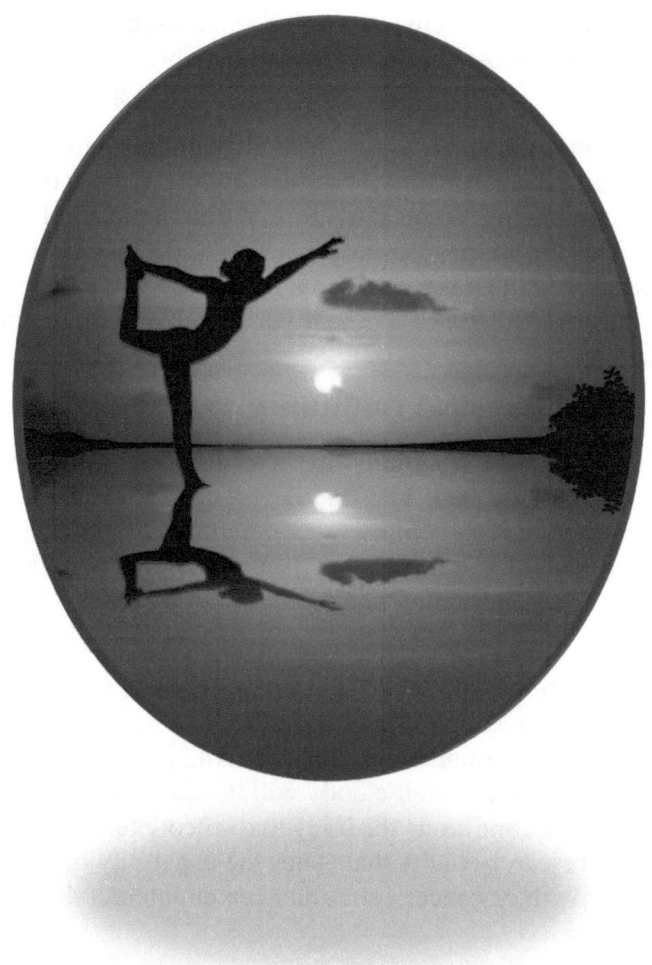

Benefits of Yoga

If you are able to determine which school fits you the most, then it is time to know what you need to expect if you are able to maintain your yoga practice. The items that will be discussed though are limited only to the most common results that a practitioner can experience.

You need also to remember as you read through this part of the book that additional results may vary depending on your reasons and goals in practicing Yoga. Therefore, if you do not find what you are looking for in this chapter since it is quite specific basing on your needs you must not be discouraged since you can still achieve it through the use of Yoga, if you are able to maintain your determination.

A. Increase Physical Immunity

Yoga will boost a person's immunity in terms of the discipline it imposes to the practitioner. The Buddhist Yoga for example teaches mostly the way of eating healthy food in contrast of undisciplined food intake. A healthy diet plan then is implemented allowing the body to increase its immunity against common diseases.

The physical exercises of yoga as well create a good body condition allowing each internal organ to function more properly. It also triggers a healthy sweating allowing the body to regulate its temperature better throughout the session. And if the proper practice is maintained, then the body will be able to adapt more to different physical conditions the body may encounter. There are even medical researches now that states the capability of Yoga to prevent the growth of cancer cells and even counteract the early stages of cancer.

B. Boost Sexual Performance

This can be related directly to the improved physical performance that Yoga presents to the practitioner. And since Yoga is a discipline that teaches you how to channel your energy properly as well, sexual performance can then be prolonged basing on the capabilities of utilizing your energy properly.

This result can also be related to the fact that Yoga can teach you the isolation of your thoughts in a single act and improve concentration while doing a specific action. The Yoga postures as well can be utilized if you prefer a more experimental approach in your sexual experience. Setting humor aside though, a good practitioner of Yoga can technically use the teachings to achieve better satisfaction in sexual performance since the body; the spirit and the mind will be working together to achieve the goal.

C. Better Recuperation

The healing process of Yoga practitioners can be faster and better than non-practitioners. The evidence for this is still the fact that Yoga diesoline demands proper diet and physical management. This triggers the body to be able to heal properly with far less effort since its energy will not be put to waste. Excess energy will be saved within the body for the purpose of using it in some other activity once the healing process is complete. Non-practitioners on the other hand may waste more energy during the healing process since their body will not be able to channel the energy properly and concentrate in the healing. Yoga enables your body to do great things, and it is only with the power of the mind that these things are possible to happen. You will feel more energized and can move around better when you are performing yoga. If you have back pains and aches, headaches or migraines or otherwise feel that you are 'stiff,' participating in yoga can turn your life around.

You must understand though that this process does not mean you will be able to heal right away through will alone. It is not magic that gives immediate results. This happens in the cellular level and is done by your body instinctively since each part of you already knows what to do and how to do it properly. It still takes time but in a more efficient way thus cutting down the time and energy that will be consumed.

D. Weight Control and Balance Metabolism

Weight control is probably the most popular goal and reason for practicing Yoga. And if you recall the previous points discussed, this goal can be achieved through the physical, mental and spiritual exercises Yoga uses. It must be emphasized once again that effort must be present especially since it involves proper diet aside from the manual labor you need to do. But if you are a true practitioner then effort is technically a second nature to you since Yoga teaches it as well.

Each Yoga posture is also designed to increase blood circulation and thus maintain good metabolism. Once you achieve this state you will also have an easier time controlling your weight since your body itself will know which condition it must maintain.

E. Increase Muscle Flexibility and Strength

Yoga poses and physical exercises are mostly the cause of stronger and more flexible muscles. Each pose will be able to stretch your muscles properly and promote better posture and thus it will adapt to increase its own strength.

Unlike other exercises that require your effort through lifting external weights, Yoga only asks you to utilize your own body to increase performance. Thus this means you will need lesser equipment as well than a normal workout in a gym.

You must set your expectation though that Yoga is not designed for bodybuilding. Its ways is to increase a balanced strength and maintain it without building too much mass. You can view it as more of toning your muscles properly than building them to be bigger.

F. Stress Management

Stress management can be done through the mental and spiritual conditioning Yoga gives to its practitioners. You will be taught how to free your mind from any emotional attachment that is burdening you through the use of meditation. You can isolate your perception to be optimistic but at the same time see everything that is happening around you. You can then broaden your insight and deal with any cause of stress you may encounter in your life. And if you will be able to maintain this state, you should be able to find enlightenment within yourself and thus will definitely live a more satisfactory life.

Again, these are not only the benefits you can achieve. You can aim for many more. It is up to you to try and reach whatever goal you may have when you start practicing Yoga. The only limit you will encounter is the boundaries you will put up yourself but Yoga will also teach you how to get rid of them.

Importance of Incorporating the Chakras

Yoga as a method of healing uses different centers of energy from within the body. When the yoga is practiced, the individual is able to gain a better awareness of them; their body, mind and soul, increasing the energy flow into the energy centers. As we have already discussed, there are a total of 7 of these chakras within the body. The chakras are responsible for awareness and are needed to keep our bodies balanced and our energy levels high.

The chakras are responsible for awareness and are needed to keep our bodies balanced and our energy levels high. The key to being successful at chakra is to bring awareness to the mind by releasing various blockages that stand in the way.

The following benefits of chakra improvement are found:

- ✓ Help eliminate hurt and pain

- ✓ Strength to carry on to another day
- ✓ Depression, anxiety treatment
- ✓ Better appetite
- ✓ Better digestion
- ✓ Improvement in relationships
- ✓ Better overall health
- ✓ More energy
- ✓ More positivity
- ✓ Add creativity and spark to your imagination

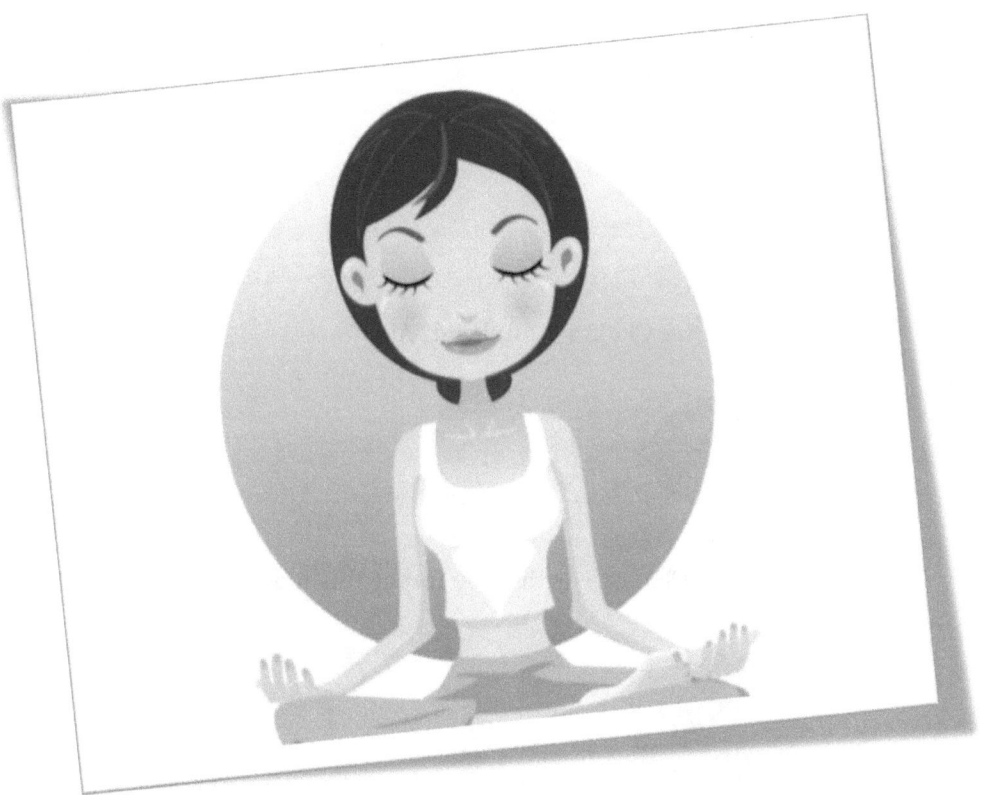

What are Chakras?

Chakras are defined as spinning wheels of electric energy within you body. The wheels are responsible for functions that connect your body to your energy field and the broader cosmic energy field.

The seven major chakras include:

- ✓ The Crown Chakra – top of the head "Sahasarara"

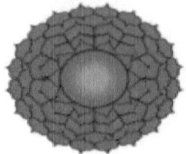

✓ The Third Eye Chakra – forehead "Ajna"

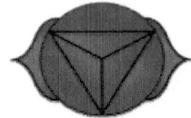

✓ The Throat Chakra – within the throat "Vishuddha"

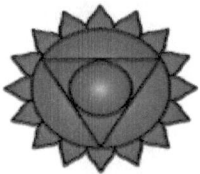

✓ The Heart Chakra – within the heart "Anahata"

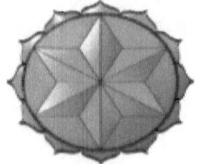

✓ The Solar Chakra – the solar plexus "Manipura"

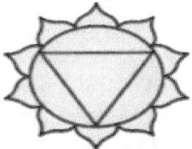

✓ The Sacral Chakra – the naval "Svadhisthana"

✓ The Root Chakra – Base of the spine "Muladhara"

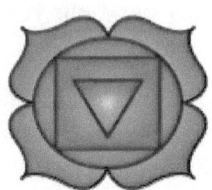

Each of the seven has their own different character and relate to one part of our life. This includes things associated with colors, the functioning of the body, elements, sounds and more. It is believed that the energy blockage that is found in the chakra is responsible to a number of different psychological and emotional disorders. It is a must that the individual have a good appreciation of the various chakras within the body. When they are not well-balanced, the individual suffers greatly.

Each of the different chakras plays a role in the way that we feel and the way that we respond to certain behaviors. It is essential just that each of the different chakras be well-balanced in order for the individual to thrive. But, that is where the problem starts. So many people in the world are not in tune with the chakras and are unable to energize themselves. They are unaware that they even exist, and when something goes wrong, like most people, they head to the physician in hopes that he can give them a remedy for their ails. While the doctor may be able to get something to you that provide temporary comfort, this is all that you will get. And, there are tons of different side affects that you also grind coming along with those doctor remedies. Furthermore you are not actually treating them when you see the doctor. Instead you are only covering them up for a period of time. This is not the way to enhance your life and it can actually cause more problems in the end. Rather than take these chances, understanding the chakras and how they can help you is a must.

The chakras are linking mechanisms between the meridian system and the auric field inside your physical body. They also serve as a connection between the different auras and the cosmic energy field. The have a major impact on the flow of energy into your body.

The word "chakra" comes from old Sanskrit. The term means "wheel" or "round," and is used to reference particular energy focuses along your bodies centerline. The very first time that chakras were mention came from Hindu scriptures. The prophets mentioned the chakras as a pillar of energy that extends from the base of the spine to the top of the head.

Your body has one hundred in twenty minor chakras to go along with the seven major chakras.

The Seven Chakras in Detail

There are a few different chakras within the body. In fact, there are seven of them. Now that you know a bit more about the Chakras, we will take a look each of the types of them and help you learn more so that changing your life and feeling better than you have ever before is something that can start as quickly as possible. We will also help you learn more about the roles that they play in the body, the affects they have when they are not in balance, and the different things that are associated with them.

"Sahasarara" The Crown Chakra – top of the head

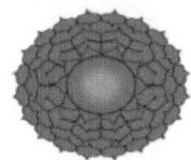

SYMBOL *"A thousand petaled lotus"*

The Sahasrara is called the thousands pedaled lotus. It is the element of thought and represents the colors white and violet. It is said to bring unity into an iniciusal and is located at the crown of the head. The mantra of the Sahasrara is at the crown of the head. This Chakra deals with the person's emotional feelings and integration of one's self. Physical dysfunctions of the Chakra include sensitivity to light and sound. The psychological issues with the Chakra include trust, apathy, ethics and materialism. When this chakra is well balanced the individual is able to maintain intelligence, is more open-minded and understanding and more easily able to adapt a variety of different information. Lotus is a related essential oil.

The crown chakra "Sahasarara" can cause a person to have difficulty thinking, a lack of concentration and a lack of empathy. Those who are not in tune with this chakra usually feel as if they are superior to other people and think that they are smarter than other people. Meditation is the most popular form of healing from this chakra. In addition to meditation, yoga and Tai chai are also beneficial.

With its location at the top of the head, the crown chakra connects to your central nervous system via the hypothalamus and the thalamus. The crown chakra governs the central nervous system, the pineal gland, the top of the head and the midline above your ears.

If this chakra is not balanced it could lead to chronic exhaustion, brain disorders, coordination problems, photosensitivity, mental sickness, epilepsy, ethics, and a lack of purpose.

"Ajna" The Third Eye Chakra – forehead between the eyes

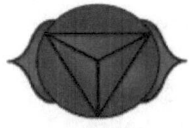

SYMBOL *"Descending triangle within a circle"*

The Ajna is the center of command. It is associated with the color indigo and is located between the eyebrows. Some people call it the third eye. This Chakra deals with the different feelings and thoughts of an individual. This includes their wisdom, intelligent level, detachment insight, understanding in, reasoning and more. This chakra, when not in balance, can cause a number of different physical attributes to occur. This includes eyestrain, difficulty learning, panic, seizures, spinal dysfunction, fear of truth, the inability to concentrate, headaches and nightmares. With a balanced Chakra it is possible to have a new reality and better concentration and focus. Mint and Jasmine help this Chakra.

The third eye, the Ajna Chakra, causes a number of different problems including those with the eyes, poor visualization, and a bad memory. It can cause a person to experience headaches on a regular basis, and even suffer with nightmares on a regular basis. Those who are deficient in this particular chakra are also prone to nightmares and hallucinating.

With its location between your eyes, the third eye chakra governs the neurological systems, the brain, pituitary gland, pineal glands, ears, nose and your eyes. The chakra has direct influence over your sense of trust, intuition and coordination. It has a direct influence over your sense of trust, intuition and coordination.

If this chakra is imbalanced you may experience issues with discipline, sleep disorders concepts of judgment and reality, emotional intelligence, confusion, blindness, stroke, seizures, brain tumors, arrogance, pride, learning disabilities and sleep disorders.

The third eye chakra enables you to put things into perspective and is key to learning and wisdom. This chakra is responsible for your intuitive intelligence and universal consciousness. Your third eye chakra helps you differentiate between reality and fantasy. When the flow of energy is blocked through this chakra, you experience a sense of distrust and self-doubt. An open and clear chakra enables you to connect with your inner wisdom and guides you in the choices you make.

"Vishuddha" The Throat Chakra – within the throat

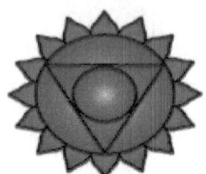

SYMBOL *"A circle within a descending triangle"*

The Vishuddha chakra is the purification chakra. It is related to the sense of hearing and is located on the nerve found in the throat near the pharynx. This chakra deals with learning abilities, responsibility for your own actions, faith, intuition and creativity. When this specific Chakra is not healed, there are many different physical complications that can arise. This includes swollen glands and gums, hearing problems, grinding of the teeth, ulcers in the mouth, swollen glands, tooth problems and more. When this chakra is balanced, as it should be, the individual is able to have positive emotions and expressions, good decision making skills, creativity and contentment. Eucalyptus and sage are the essential oils believed to benefit this particular chakra.

The throat chakra deficiency can cause fears, tension and neck stiffness. If you want to enhance this chakra it requires that you have a well balanced diet, participate in mediation on a regular basis, and of course perform yoga. Drinking water is also beneficial to those who want to energize this particular chakra. You can also do things such as shoulder openers, neck stretches and yoga poses like the Bridge Pose and the Camel Pose to benefit yourself.

With its location near your throat, the Vishuddha chakra governs the mouth, gums, teeth, trachea, thyroid, vertebrae, neck, throat, esophagus, parathyroid and hypothalamus. It directly influences your sense of security, independence, self-expressions, loyalty, communication, planning and organization.

If this chakra is out of balance, the impact could result in the flu, fever, sore throat, swollen glands, thyroid imbalance, laryngitis, scoliosis, mouth ulcers, gum problems, vocal issues, tooth problems, faith, criticism, addictions, and decision-making.

The throat chakra is the center of your will power and communication. If you struggle to make choices or decisions it stems from this energy center. It also serves as the communication center with a divine power. Your faith is based in this energy center. Your ability to communicate the truth and voice your opinions is based on the throat chakra. With a clear throat chakra you are able to express your truth without any worries of what others may think or say. If the chakra is blocked, however, it will create anxiousness about how others react to your views and this leads to restraint.

"Anahata" The Heart Chakra – within the heart

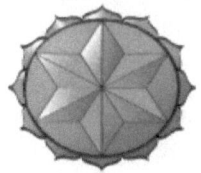

SYMBOL *"Intertwined descending and ascending triangles"*

This chakra relates to the sense of touch. It is located near the plexus of the heart and affects an individual's self-identity, their ability to provide wisdom and unconditional love, their ability to have patience and comparison. When this chakra is not balanced it affects the upper back and the shoulders, can cause asthma and heart conditions, lung diseases and the spine. There are also emotional issues that can surround an individual who is not balanced with this chakra, and this includes a lack of empathy, lack of compassion, anger and anxiety and even jealousy. When this chakra is balanced there is an empathic feeling, you are optimistic and free of resentment. Essential oils to help balance this chakra include lavender and jasmine.

This fourth chakra is the heart chakra. It separates the chakras from one another, and usually results in characteristics that affect an individual's way of spirit. Those who are defiance in this area are oftentimes shy and lack empathy. They do not forgive easily and oftentimes are anger and unable to form good connections with other people. There are a number of negative health effects that can result from this deficiency, including problems with, what else, the heart? Common problems include high blood pressure, heart disease and jealousy. To work on this chakra, yoga poses are recommended, including backbends and the Eagle Pose. While these things are beneficial, it is loving and the ability to do that that helps the most and offers the most powerful form of rehabilitation.

With its location at the center of your chest, the Anahata chakra governs the lungs, blood, circulatory system, thymus, diaphragm, heart, esophagus, shoulders, arms, legs and breast.

The heart chakra has a direct influence over compassion, forgiveness, passion, devotion, love for self, love for others, and your circulatory system. If this chakra is unbalanced, it can lead to issues like lung cancer, pneumonia, breast cancer, shoulder problems, confidence issues, envy, fear, hate, despair, confidence, passivity and jealousy.

The heart chakra is a storehouse of your energy system and the center of healing and love. This energy center is connected to your emotions and empowers you to give and love unconditionally. It also facilitates any emotional healing that is required and serves as a connection between your body and soul. You will feel connected to everyone in your life when this chakra is open and flowing.

"Manipura" The Solar Chakra – the solar plexus

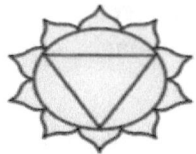

SYMBOL *"Descending triangle"*

The Manipura is the element of fire. It is related to the sense of color and sight. This chakra is found on the gastric or the solar plexus region of the umbilicus. This chakra affects the person's sense of well-being, their ability to understand and deal with emotional problems, stamina and the willpower and ego of an individual. There are a number of consequences of an unbalanced Manipura charka. Those include diabetes, arthritis, stomach pain and stomach ulcers, low blood pressure, lack of self esteem, depression, inability to make decisions, hostility and poor decision making abilities. Some people also experience anger and bouts of rage. With a balanced chakra there is a great amount of energy, and the person is left with confidence and intelligence to make good decisions. This chakra, when well balanced, allows for positive mental focus, good digestive health and better productivity throughout the day. Rosemary and lavender are among the essential oils that are said to enhance this chakra.

The Solar Plexus, or Manipura Chakra, causes a number of emotional problems such as low self-esteem, bad self-image and no energy. It can also cause anger, the need to be more powerful than another person and the need to be perfect and all ways. This can cause depression to develop as well as the person to need stimulants. Yoga is especially helpful for this third chakra, and participating in techniques such as the Half Boat Pose, Leg Lifts and the Boat Pose are all beneficial.

Located just above the navel, this chakra governs the upper abdomen, liver, pancreas, middle spine, gall bladder, adrenals, kidney, spleen, stomach, and the small intestine.

The chakra influences your self-confidence, growth, self-control, humor, self-power, ego power and digestion. If this chakra is imbalanced it may result in diabetes, constipation, digestive problems, ulcers, self-esteem issues, oversensitivity to criticism, self-image fears, nervousness and poor memory.

The Manipura chakra defines your self-esteem. Your mental awareness, ego, optimism, will power and confidence originate from your solar plexus chakra. The chakra is the energy center that rules your concentration power and your ability to comprehend things. Your natural instincts flow through this chakra.

"Svadhisthana" The Sacral Chakra – the naval

SYMBOL *"Up-turned crescent"*

This chakra is the element of water and deals with the individual's ability to taste. It is found between the genitals and the sacral plexus nerve. This chakra deals with emotions, creativity and pleasure of personal relationships. It governs the liver and gallbladder, the stomach and kidneys and the adrenal glands. When there is an imbalance in this chakra there is lower back pain, problems with digestion, menstrual cycle problems, hormonal imbalances, pelvic pain, feelings of being tired and problems with psychological concerns such as money, power and a lack of creativity. Those who have this chakra in balance are compassionate, satisfied with their sexual being, prosperous and humorous. The Amber and Orange Tourmaline gemstones are related to this chakra, as is the Sandalwood and Ylang-Ylang essential oils.

This chakra is responsible for your sensual and emotional well-being. When there is sacral deficiency there are many different problems that may manifest, which can include fertility issues, fears of change and even problems becoming intimate with other people. When there is a deficiency here there is oftentimes an exhibit of extreme emotional behavior. When you use the simple forms of yoga you can enhance the sacral chakra. You can do a variety of yoga poses to help here, and usually it is nothing more than a bit of gentle stretching that causes powerful sensations to be empowered to you. In addition to yoga, listening to music and aromatherapy are beneficial in this department.

With its location below your navel in your lower abdomen, the chakra governs the sexual organs, gonad gland, liver, stomach, gall bladder, kidney, upper intestine, adrenal glands, spleen and middle spine. It plays a major influence on joyfulness, enthusiasm, reproduction, and creativity.

If this chakra is imbalanced, anger issues may occur, apathy, hatred, menace, greed, guilt, control, power, immortality, pelvic pain, gynecological problems, urinary problems and libido issues.

The Svadhisthana is your creative center. It has influence in you finances, personal power, and your sexual center. This energy center connects you to your inner child, your feelings, and sensualities. It is tied to physical feelings of passion, love and sexuality. This chakra also facilitates the act of giving and receiving.

"Muladhara" The Root Chakra – Base of the spine

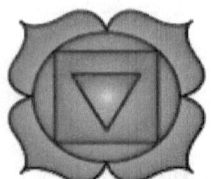

SYMBOL *"Square with a descending triangle"*

Muladhara is the element of the earth and affects the smell. It is found in between the genitals and the anus along the base of the spine. It deals with ambition, self-sufficiency, and stability, and governs the teeth, kidneys and sexual activity. Those with an imbalance in this chakra oftentimes suffer from poor sleeping habits, lower back pain, problems with waste elimination including constipation, being tired all of the time, anger, low self esteem, feeling alienated or possessive. When this chakra is balanced there is a feeling of independence, vitality and energy. Foods are digested much easier and you are overall much happier. The Ruby is a gemstone related to this chakra, and the cedar and clove are the related essential oils.

If you are deficient in the Muladhara, or root chakra, insecurities abound. This can be anything from money troubles to relationship problems that cause you to become insecure. When this happens you are probably feeling empty and lost inside, and anxiety creeps up on a continuous basis. There are even symptoms that can cause an individual to start hoarding and cause weight gain. If you want to help alleviate the problems that come with an unbalanced root chakra, one of the best things that you can do is a leg move during your yoga. Stretching the hamstring can once again balance the root chakra. There are many different standing yoga poses that can help you do this, and they also promote patience and calmness, so healing yourself mentally and physically is possible.

The root chakra governs the reproductive organs, the spinal cord, immune system, adrenal glands, rectum, and the legs and feet. It has a direct influence over your mental stability, sense of security, sensuality, and sexuality. If the chakra is not balanced, it could result in varicose veins, lower back pain, depression, immunity related disorders, rectal tumors, low self-esteem, and security issues.

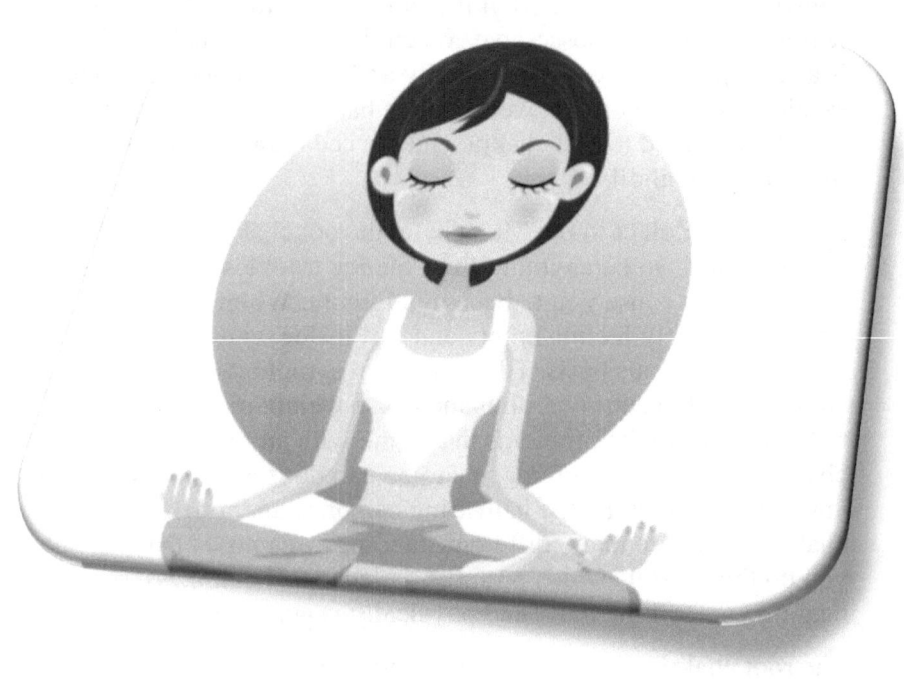

Yoga Equipment for Beginners

You are now ready to prepare yourself for the first Yoga session you will attend. And as what was mentioned in the previous chapter, Yoga exercises do not demand too much use of equipment since most poses and forms utilizes your own body.

The equipment that will be discussed is the most basic that a yoga practitioner needs. As a matter of fact, the equipment may the only ones you will ever use throughout all your sessions. You need to remember though that it is not necessary for you to buy all of these since if you are attending a Yoga school they most probably have almost all of the equipment that will be mentioned.

If you take a look at the items listed below as well, you will see that most of them can be improvised by using available items you have at home. But that only would be the case if you prefer to have sessions within your home as well using the simple guide this book will be giving you in the next two chapters. Still, it would be best to seek out guidance for your first few sessions from a Yoga Guru that can give you additional information that you might need.

A. Clothing and Outfit

There are no special outfits that a Yoga practitioner must wear while doing Yoga. Normal gym clothes are actually enough for you to be able to move freely and do the poses and forms with little to no obstruction at all.

What you must remember though when choosing the gym clothes is the comfort they provide you. Do not wear those clothes designed to make you sweat even more if you think that it will allow you to lose weight even faster. It won't work the way you want it to since it will compromise the concentration and focus Yoga wants you to have with each session. Just ensure that your clothes will have a good fit, not too tight, not too loose. The fabric must also be stretchable enough to allow maximum movement and flexibility.

Some Yoga schools though may require you to wear specific clothing especially for meditations but that seldom happens especially if you are with a Modern Yoga School.

B. Yoga Mat

A Yoga mat is the equipment that you can use to provide comfort each time you do a pose or a form in your sessions. There are actually multiple types of mats in the market that can be utilize not only for Yoga but also with other forms of exercise. They differ in sizes as well from as small as only a single person can use or as large as an entire room.

Most schools though already provide these mats for the practitioners making it one less equipment you really need to buy. Other schools may also not require you to use a mat depending on the culture and tradition the school follows.

C. Yoga Blanket

A yoga blanket like the yoga mat provides comfort for every session you do. Technically speaking you will no longer need to use this one if you already have a mat. But sometimes you might want to have an extra cushion under you each time you strike a pose or form. The use of the blanket may also vary depending on the school.

A normal blanket can actually replace a yoga blanket as long as the blanket is just large enough for one person to use. You do not want any excess fabric distracting you and hindering your movement.

D. Yoga Blocks

Yoga blocks are used generally for support especially if the practitioner is not yet flexible enough to perform a specific post or form. It can then become very useful for a beginner since it lessen the effort you would need to exert for a pose but will still give you maximum output and result.

Even advance Yoga practitioners utilize these blocks upon performing really complex forms for the first time. This essentially makes you adapt to the posture until your body is capable enough to support itself without the assistance of the blocks. Try to think about them as the training wheels of a bicycle but instead of making you ride them, you will be stationary and worry less that you might fall.

There are poses and forms though that will not require a Yoga block even if you are just a beginner just like most of the forms in the next two chapters.

E. Yoga Straps

Similar to Yoga blocks, Yoga straps are used mainly for practitioners who still have less flexibility. As the name implies, the straps are tied to a specific body part and then pulled by the user to reach the maximum flexibility the body can handle without injury. It will help you to hold the position you are performing within the time you would need to strike the pose. It is then very useful if your body is still incapable to holding itself still especially for forms you are doing the first time.

Take note though that you need to feel the limit of your body each time you use the straps. Others may think that pulling it further beyond the limit may hasten the improvement of body flexibility. But if you are not careful and force your body too much, the strap may cause injury, which will counteract the true purpose of performing a Yoga form. The good thing though, unlike most of the other exercise equipment, the Yoga strap is controlled by your own force and does not have any additional weight that can affect its influence over your body. You can let go of it any time you want once you feel your body could no longer take the pressure.

F. Why Shoes are Unnecessary

For a beginner, you might start to think while the shoes are never mentioned since the Table of contents of the book. Well, you do not really need to wear one while practicing Yoga.

The main reason why you do not need any shoes for a Yoga session is the fact that you are not going to use them in any pose or form Yoga will ask you to perform. You will not be moving most of the time and thus not really need to protect your feet as if you are using the treadmill or jogging around a course. At most, shoes can only serve as a distraction while you are performing poses that involve the full use of your feet and you toes. Most Yoga schools will also require you to remove them once the session starts.

The equipments are of course just a small part of the entire routine. And as you notice, almost all of them are designed to either give comfort or support. As you progress in your Yoga practice, you might not even need to use some of the equipment. Investing in your personal equipment then is not really necessary especially if you do not pane to practice Yoga at home.

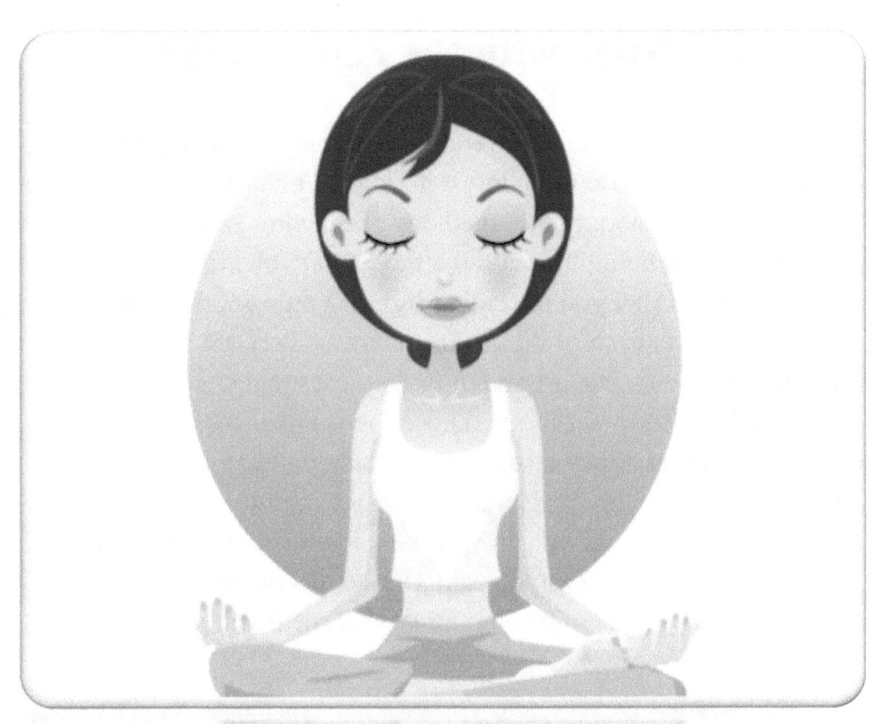

Enhance Yoga with the right Foods

We have talked about the different ways that you can enhance the chakras, with a particular interest in yoga to enhance them. But, we have also talked about other methods of opening and empowering the chakras, including through the foods that you are consuming. It is so important that you are eating right if you want the best connection with each of the seven chakras. There are so many different nutrients that are found in the foods that we consume, when they are the right foods. Those foods enhance the brainpower that you have, and they also affect the way that you will feel. Let's examine some of the foods that you might want to consume to enhance your chakras. It is in your best interest to add as many of these foods to the diet as you can. There are a number of different ways that this can be done no matter what meal that you are trying to cover.

As we have already stated it is important that you are eating a colorful meal. The more colorful the plate, the healthier that it is, and the more advancement that you can do for your chakras. Each chakra is related to a color. Make sure that you are eating foods that contain all of these colors.

Important to remember when eating to enhance the chakras: no meat. If you are eating an animal you are promoting killing and other acts of violence. The entire purpose of chakra healing is to avoid negativity and bad karma. If you are eating animals you are certainly not using the power of the chakras. Rather than eating animals and meat, there are many healthy fruits and vegetables that you can consume to complete the diet. You will still get the needed protein in your body and also adhere fully to the power of the chakra and self-awareness of them.

Also keep in mind that it is oftentimes the root chakra that is the most essential in eating the right foods. There are so many problems that are caused at the root chakra, and without this well-balanced meal, there are a number of effects that can result. When you change your diet to include foods that are beneficial to the chakra, this is not a problem that you will experience. Colorful foods are best to enhance the root chakra. This includes red foods, with a particular interest in fruits and berries of this color. Root vegetables are also highly recommended, including yam. The chakra is a part of the earth. Foods that are symbolic with the earth and the soil are good foods that you want to include in the menu. Mushrooms are another excellent choice that can be enjoyed on a regular basis to enhance the senses of the chakra. The mushrooms are packed with protein and are from the soil, both of which you want.

Take a look at these favorite foods that you should enjoy to enhance the chakras. You're sure to find a variety of ways to introduce them into your diet, and you'll love them all!

1. **Pomegranate:** Pomegranate is another root chakra beneficial food that you can enjoy. This sweet fruit heightens all of the senses and tastes great!
2. **Oranges:** Another root chakra food beneficial to consume – oranges. What you might not know about oranges is that they can excite the chakras and all of your sexual desire and energy. So in addition to adding an enormous amount of vitamin C to your body, eating an orange will enhance your chakra and might very well cause a little bit of excitement in the bedroom.

3. **Corn on the Cob:** Corn on the cob is another yellow specialty that will enhance yoga and your chakras. Enjoy it as a nice side item with your favorite entrée.
4. **Spinach:** Spinach is a green, leafy vegetable with plenty of vitamins and minerals inside of it. Along with those qualities, spinach is also beneficial in enhancing the third chakra. With this enhancement you will learn better communication methods and will feel more positive each day.
5. **Yellow Peppers:** These peppers enhance the flavors of foods, but they do so much more, too. They can improve the functioning of your pancreas, which in turn also helps you with self-worth, your instincts, and more. Some people refer to this chakra as the third brain. Add yellow peppers to the menu as often as possible.
6. **Kale:** kale is another veggie to be included on the menu. This particular vegetable is beneficial to the heart chakra and helps the person feel love, empathy and similar emotions that we all need to feel. Kale can be combined with so many different meals, and provides an outstanding number of health benefits as well as a great way to improve the heart chakra energy and promote your well-being.
7. **Blueberries:** Rich in antioxidants, blueberries are the go-to snack when you want to enhance your third eye chakra. Regular blueberry consumption will give you a great boost of energy and help you mentally, too.
8. **Beets:** This red vegetable can be served raw or cooked, and offers a sweet taste that can satisfy your hunger. It is fiber-rich and high in antioxidants and enables energy to freely flow from the chakras.
9. **Nuts:** Nuts benefit yoga greatly, and like most of the other foods that we have listed here are beneficial to the health in many other ways. They are a great snack that can be enjoyed at home or on the go, paced with protein that can fuel you for the day. Make sure that you have your favorite nuts (excluding peanutso readily available at all times.

10. **Water:** Our body is made up of nearly 70% water, so, as you might suspect, you need it for proper bodily function. It is recommended that adults consume no less than eight glasses of H2O each day. This amount should be enough to suffice for what you lose in a single day. Water is lost from the body through numerous functions, including sweating and urination. Make sure that you replace that water and you will look better and you feel better too. There is nothing in this world that is healthier than water, so choose it any time that you need a great thirst quencher.

Your body needs a wide variety of raw foods to thrive properly. The 10 listed above are among the best choices that you have when you want to enhance the energy that is found within the chakras, but this is only a sampling of the things that you can enjoy to enhance your chakras. Along with taking all of the other measures of improving the energy that flows to the chakra, make sure that you are also carefully monitoring the foods that you are eating. When it is a well-balanced diet that you are eating on a regular basis, then you can be sure that you are getting what you need in your body. It can start with these foods. They are great for you to consume in more ways than one, certain to bring you into the energizing state that you desire to be in.

Yoga Poses for Beginners Part 1

It is now time to learn a few forms in Yoga that can be done by beginners. Each post is also designed for those who are not that flexible yet. The benefits of the poses will also be given to allow you to understand why each post must be performed properly.

A. The Mountain

Use: The mountain or Tadasana is a form the can be used as a breathing exercise. It will also improve your posture and sense of center.

Form: To perform the mountain all you need to do is stand up straight with your feet spread hip-width apart. Align your neck straight to your spine and then breathe slowly in a constant pace. You can stretch out your arms up to increase flexibility or assume a prayer position to improve focus.

B. The Dog facing Down

Use: Adho Mukha Svansana is used to improve the overall body circulation. It also stretches the calves and heels of the practitioner.

Form: Keep your feet hip width apart and slowly bend over to allow both of your hands to touch the ground creating an arc on your body. You must do this while keeping your feet flat to the ground. Walk your hands forward a little until your arms, shoulders and back are aligned. The arms should be shoulder width apart. If you are using a mat for a single person use, your fingers must reach near the front of the mat and your toes near the rear of the mat. Keep your fingers spread for added support.

C. The Dog facing Up

Use: Urdhava Mukha Svansana's main purpose is to stretch your spine, wrists and arms.

Form: Lie facing down on your mat and keep your two thumbs under your shoulders. Extend your legs straight and keep your ankles facing up. Secure your hips on the mat then start pushing your chest upwards while keeping your shoulders down. Look up and hold for a few seconds. Then slowly go back to the starting position of the post and relax. Then repeat the process.

D. The Warrior

Use: The Virabhadrasana is good for stretching your leg and ankles as well as increasing their strengths.

Form: Stand with your legs at least four feet apart. Turn your right foot ninety degrees to the right and your left foot slightly following the direction the right foot is pointing. Extend your arms to your side at shoulder level and keep your palms facing down. Bend your right knee at ninety degrees and slightly lunge your other knee to compensate for support. Do not let your right knee extend beyond your right foot. Repeat the process on the other foot.

E. The Tree

Use: The mountain or Vriksasana is can be used to improve your balance by strengthening your thighs, calves, ankle and spine.

Form: Stand straight on one leg and bring the other ankle up to the standing leg as high as possible depending on how flexible you are. If you are still not able to support your weight with one leg, you can lean with your back flat on a wall. Raise your hands and assume a prayer position with palms above your head to for a posture similar to a tree. Remember to repeat the same position but use the other leg as support to develop both legs at the same time.

Yoga Poses for Beginners Part 2

In this chapter are four more poses a beginner can use. Remember that with each form you need to breathe regularly and properly to keep your focus and meditation.

A. The Bridge

Use: Setu Bhanda will strengthen your chest, neck, and spine. You can also use this as a good warm-up for harder back bends.

Form: Lie down back flat on the floor with your hands on the side. Bend your knees and keep both feet on the floor. Slowly lift your hips and press your arms down for support. Keep your hips parallel to the mat as you try to press your chest near your chin. You can also put a pillow under your chest or head if you are not yet flexible enough.

B. The Triangle

Use: Trikonasana or the triangle can relieve backaches by strengthening your thighs, knees and ankles.

Form: Do the warrior post but this time; do not lunge with your knee to form the ninety-degree angle. Then place the back of your right hand on your right foot without bending your knees. Then raise your left hand and point all its fingers towards the ceiling. Repeat the process on the other foot.

C. The Pigeon

Use: The Eka pada Rajakapotsana stretches your quads by opening up your shoulders and chests.

Form: Do the push up position with your palms under your shoulder. Then bring your right knee near your right shoulder, keep the heel near your hip. Press up with your arms keeping your chest out. Sit on your right leg and hold the position. Repeat the process using the other leg.

D. The Child

Use: The Balasana allows you to relax while stretching your hips, thighs and ankles.

Form: Start by kneeling with both knees and lower legs flat on the floor, your ankles and heels must be facing upward. Then sit on your legs and spread your knees a little. You can now rest your belly between the knees and stretch your hands straight over your head with both palms on the mat.

Yoga: Let's Get Started

While it would be nice if you could simply pop in an instructional video and learn how to do yoga this is not the way that you want to learn how to do things. Yes, it is an option and there are many people who do this rather than ever making a visit to a yoga studio. Not only are you causing yourself potential injury and damage by trying to take things into your own hands, you might also face the trouble of learning improper techniques, the last thing that you want to happen as you are trying to advance yourself and the life that you are liking. This is just the start of the many dangers that can come along with trying to learn yoga on your own.

Now, if you want to make the purchase of one of those DVDs hat teach you yoga from the comfort of your home, this is an option that is available to you. But why would you want to cause potential damage to your life when you are trying to make great changes? Someone, somewhere, is looking to make money off of you through these DVDs. But, this is probably not the option that you want to choose, especially if you are new to the world of yoga. Not only do you need a certified yoga instructor to teach you how to do things so that you are not injuring yourself or hurting your body, it is also important that you are able to mentally connect with the chakra so that you can benefit, as you should be from doing yoga.

Finding a Yoga Instructor

Hatha is the most commonly chosen type of yoga performed by beginners and individuals who are ready to tune into their energy and chakras. It enlists the basic yoga moves and helps familiarize the individual with the techniques and the various moves. We all know that yoga can take time to master, thus starting off with this form is an excellent idea. Of course, if you prefer to do something else it is completely up to you, nut it is important that you are aware of the types that are out there, and the one that you want to do. Not all yoga instructors or studios offer the same type of instruction, thus making sure of what you want and what you are getting ahead of time is a must.

There are many ways to research the various types of yoga out there, as well as their benefits and how they can help you regain the lost energy with the chakras. This includes using the Internet, looking inside of history journals and publications and of course through research papers. Yoga has a very interesting history, and dates back for centuries in Chinese medicine. It is very interesting to learn and it can help you out as you advance.

Make sure that you take the time to visit the website of any instructor that you are considering. On the website you can learn a wide variety of information about the center, including the year that it started and the different types of yoga that they are offering to the world. You might also want to use the web to find reviews of the center from people who have firsthand experience using the company. There are various websites that offer testimonials and other information about the yoga instruction, and with this information you can benefit yourself greatly.

Next, research the various yoga studios near your. Most people choose a center that is close in proximity to work or school since this makes thing sore convenient. However, you are always free to choose where you will go for yoga. While you are searching for studios in your area, make sure that you are also getting to know more about them through the same resources as mentioned above.

You do not want to trust your alternative health means to just anyone, and with so many different resource to help you, there is no reason to do so.

What should you seek to find when choosing your yoga studio? It is far more than the convenient location (which, of course, we hope that you are able to find.)

You must also take the time to learn yoga etiquette. It is very important to familiar yourself with this so you won't feel so out of place while in class and also to give yourself an advantage to some of the others. The etiquette of yoga must be followed with each class. It is all a part of freeing yourself, your body, mind and soul.

The cost of the class is another concern that many people have, and yet another reason that comparing is so important to do. Not all classes will cost the same amount of money; so if you are worried about this at all, make sure that you are aware of the prices ahead of time. Most studios have their prices listed on their website if you take a look. If you are not on the web or prefer to speak to someone in person, this is also possible and they will be more than happy to inform you of the prices that you will pay for the specifics that you are interested in.

It is very important that you take your classes and the instruction very seriously. Yoga is not for the weak hearted and must be followed precisely for the full benefits to result. It is for those who truly want to change their mind and become in tune with their inner being.

Tips for Success

Once you have made the decision to perform yoga and have chosen the studio that will help teach you, a few other things are in store for you to learn in order to fully benefit with your new found teachings.

First, as we have mentioned countless times throughout this life, you need to be in tune with your body, as well as your mind. Some of the moves and positions of yoga are not for the light-hearted, as they stretch your body in ways that you might not have even realized possible for the body to move.

Have you purchased an outfit that is designed especially for participation in yoga? It is necessary that you are wearing clothing that is comfortable and easy on the body, and while it may not necessarily be the yoga outfit that you want to wear, they are a lot of fun to purchase.

While you are out shopping, choose a mat. The yoga mat is a very important piece of the puzzle of success. You want to be as comfortable as you possibly can as you are performing the various techniques of yoga, and it's with the mat and the comfortable yoga type clothing that you are wearing that will make a world of difference in things. Many different types of mats are available for yoga. They are made of various materials and constructed of various sizes. One of the mats can be purchased at an affordable price, and you want to make sure that you are choosing a good mat. Again, your entire experience with yoga is dependent upon a nice, comfortable mat and the clothing that you are wearing.

There is no way for you to know just what to do during the first few classes. So, it is okay to look and to listen, but make sure that you are trying. Take special note of the alignment of the instructor. This is one of the first things that must be done in order to c conquer yoga. As you are looking at other people and observing what they are doing you will begin to pick up on things and better learn how to do yoga.

Finally, make sure that you take things slowly and never try to rush. Anything worth having taken time to achieve, and you should not expect those great changes to be made in a night or even in a week. The more that you are participating the easier that things will become, and before you know it, a yoga pro you will be! As long as you have patience and the eagerness and desire to success you can certainly do just that! No matter who you are, what type of background you come from or the ideal results that you want, they can be found!

Opening the Chakras

Just as you start participating in yoga, opening the chakras is a process that must be taken slowly. It is not something that you will fully grasp in a single night, nor is it something that should be expected. Understanding that there are chakras, and that you want to change your overall being, is the first step in identifying and connecting with the chakras that are within you.

To open the chakras that you have it is important that you discard all of the distrust that you may have, and that you are able to form a connection mentally. The first chakra is the red chakra, or the root chakra. This is the root chakra because it is the one that is responsible for helping you become aware of yourself and your mental state.

You will need to determine the ways that you will open the chakra as well. This guide has presented you with the many different ways that this can be done. It is important that you focus on each of them and ensure that you are prepared. You must be willing to do them all in order to attain the best amount of success possible. As we have mentioned time and time again, yoga is one of the very best ways that you can become in tune with the seven chakras that are found within your body.

It is usually with the help of your instructor that you learn the best ways of becoming in tune with your chakras. For most people it takes years and years of practice in order to be able to gain a full sense of wellbeing with the chakras. Once you have gained the proper instruction and have begun to feel energized through the different chakras it is then that you may be able to start doing things on your own.

Learning your chakras, as well as how to become in tune with them, is certainly a life changing experience. It can change your entire persona, the whole person that you are. It isn't for those who aren't truly focused upon arraigning success however; so make sure that you are committed from the start.

As you learn the different chakras and yoga techniques to perform them you will be able to become a new you, the person that you always wanted to be, the person that you knew was there but did not know how to break out. It is something that can now be done if you can connect to yourself body, mind and soul.

Finding The Right Yoga Instructor

Hatha is the most commonly chosen type of yoga performed by beginners and individuals who are ready to tune into their energy and chakras. It enlists the basic yoga moves and helps familiarize the individual with the techniques and the various moves. We all know that yoga can take time to master, thus starting off with this form is an excellent idea. Of course, if you prefer to do something else it is completely up to you, but it is important that you are aware of the types that are out there, and the one that you want to do. Not all yoga instructors or studios offer the same type of instruction, thus making sure of what you want and what you are getting ahead of time is a must.

There are many ways to research the various types of yoga out there, as well as their benefits and how they can help you regain the lost energy with the chakras. This includes using the Internet, researching history journals and publications and of course through research papers. Yoga has a very interesting history, and dates back for centuries in Chinese medicine. It is very interesting to learn and it can help you out as you advance.

Make sure that you take the time to visit the website of any instructor that you are considering. On the website you can learn a wide variety of information about the center, including the year that it started and the different types of yoga that they are offering to the world. You might also want to use the web to find reviews of the center from people who have firsthand experience using the company. There are various websites that offer testimonials and other information about the yoga instruction, and with this information you can benefit yourself greatly.

Next, research the various yoga studios near your. Most people choose a center that is close in proximity to work or school since this makes thing sore convenient. However, you are always free to choose where you will go for yoga. While you are searching for studios in your area, make sure that you are also getting to know more about them through the same resources as mentioned above. You do not want to trust your alternative health means to just anyone, and with so many different resource to help you, there is no reason to do so.

What should you seek to find when choosing your yoga studio? It is far more than the convenient location (which, of course, we hope that you are able to find.)

You must also take the time to learn yoga etiquette. It is very important to familiar yourself with this so you won't feel so out of place while in class and also to give yourself an advantage to some of the others. The etiquette of yoga must be followed with each class. It is all a part of freeing yourself; body, mind and soul.

The cost of the class is another concern that many people have, and yet another reason that comparing is so important to do. Not all classes will cost the same amount of money; so if you are worried about this at all, make sure that you are aware of the prices ahead of time. Most studios have their prices listed on their website if you take a look. If you are not on the web or prefer to speak to someone in person, this is also possible and they will be more than happy to inform you of the prices that you will pay for the specifics that you are interested in.

It is very important that you take your classes and the instruction very seriously. Yoga is not for the weak hearted and must be followed precisely for the full benefits to result. It is for those who truly want to change their mind and become in tune with their inner being.

The Final Word

Thank you again for downloading this book!

Studying Yoga is a good way for you to relax and achieve a peaceful mind with all the meditation practices it will impart. But not knowing the necessary information will not give you the desired results. Since you were able to finish this book you should be well equipped with at least the most basic of the information a beginner should have.

The information given to you should be able to jump-start you in your practice of Yoga. Keep in mind all the basic knowledge given to you and try to get a feel of yourself if this is really the best exercise routine that you need. Do not forget the purposes of Yoga as well. And remember, the ultimate goal is to achieve nirvana. It may take time to reach that stage but as you perceiver with your Yoga, then it is not impossible for you to reach this goal.

Finally, if you enjoyed this book, then I'd like to ask you for a favor, would you be kind enough to leave a review for this book on Amazon? It'd be greatly appreciated!

required to render accounting, officially permitted, or otherwise, qualified services. If advice is necessary, legal or professional, a practiced individual in the profession should be ordered.

- From a Declaration of Principles which was accepted and approved equally by a Committee of the American Bar Association and a Committee of Publishers and Associations.

within this book are for clarifying purposes only and are the owned by the owners themselves, not affiliated with this document.

Disclaimer

Legal Notice: - The author and publisher of this book and the accompanying materials have used their best efforts in preparing the material. The author and publisher make no representation or warranties with respect to the accuracy, applicability, fitness or completeness of the contents of this book. The information contained in this book is strictly for educational purposes. Therefore, if you wish to apply ideas contained in this book, you are taking full responsibility for your actions.

The author and publisher disclaim any warranties (express or implied), merchantability, or fitness for any particular purpose. The author and publisher shall in no event be held liable to any party for any direct, indirect, punitive, special, incidental or other consequential damages arising directly or indirectly from any use of this material, which is provided "as is", and without warranties.

As always, the advice of a competent legal, tax, accounting or other professional should be sought. The author and publisher do not warrant the performance, effectiveness or applicability of any sites listed or linked to in this book. All links are for information purposes only and are not warranted for content, accuracy or any other implied or explicit purpose.